Yoga

for

Stress Relief

And

Forgiveness

Lisa Shea

Content copyright © 2015 by

Lisa Shea / Minerva Webworks LLC

All rights reserved

No part of this book may be reproduced in any form or by any electronic or mechanical means including information storage and retrieval systems, without permission in writing from the author. The only exception is by a reviewer, who may quote short excerpts in a review.

~ v9 ~

Kindle ASIN: B00S75ILFQ

Lulu ISBN: 978-1-312-82779-0

SmashWords ISBN: 9781310020469

Note: I am not a doctor. Please always consult with your medical doctor before embarking on any exercise routine. Always listen to your body and stop if you feel any pain or discomfort.

The ebook version of this should be free in all formats and on all systems. If you buy the paperback version, or get it from a system which is not currently free, all author's proceeds are donated to battered women's shelters.

INTRODUCTION

The word "yoga" in Sanskrit means *listen*. Listening is the key to what yoga is all about. It is about listening to your body. Stretching, bending, breathing, and listening. It's about becoming more aware of your body, its strengths, where it needs help, and nurturing it.

I am a practitioner of the Kripalu style of yoga. Named after Swami Kripalu, this style emphasizes gentle, loving kindness to your body, forgiveness to your heart, and listening to what your body is telling you. You don't have to twist yourself into a pretzel. You don't have to out-do or even match the person next to you. All you have to do is take care of yourself, in whatever way is appropriate for you today.

Take it one step at a time.

Yoga is proven, by study after study, to help with body health. A 2011 study by the National Institute of Health found that yoga alleviated chronic lower back pain. A study done by Harvard found that yoga helped lift depression, even more so than other gentle forms of exercise like walking. Researchers at the trauma center of JRI find that yoga helps with post-traumatic stress disorder.

Johns Hopkins University found that yoga helps build balance, even in seniors for whom falling can be a serious issue. A study by the University of South Carolina found that yoga reduces blood pressure.

My yoga practice focuses on stress relief and forgiveness. Both are just so important in being able to focus and thrive. Each day we have is a gift. It is a blessing that we should treasure. By having the most focus we can, the least stress, and the most positive energy to apply to our own tasks and to share with the world, we make the most of that gift.

Namaste.

Note: I am not a doctor. Please always consult with your medical doctor before embarking on any exercise routine. Always listen to your body and stop if you feel any pain or discomfort.

Yoga should *not hurt*. Yoga is about gentle stretching and holding. If something hurts, you should stop. It could be you are pushing your body too hard for its current strengths. It could be something about the specific position simply does not work well given an injury or other situation with your body. There should never be pain. There should be gentle stretching.

For me, yoga is intensely pleasurable. It feels wonderful to press into the spinal twists – as if I'm receiving an expert massage. Lowering down from bridge, vertebrae by vertebrae, is sheer bliss. I've heard from many other yoga practitioners that they feel the same way. So that is something to look forward to, if you're just getting started!

The ebook version of this content should be free in all formats and on all systems. If you buy the paperback version, or get it from a system which is not currently free, all author's proceeds are donated to battered women's shelters.

ABOUT KRIPALU YOGA

I could easily write a massive tome about the history of yoga and the many branches of styles. I'll keep this brief, because the book's focus is on my personal routine, not on a history spanning thousands of years. Still, I think it's good for a person to have an inkling of what they are doing.

Yoga's roots began in India in around 500BC. To simplify, it is about helping your mind focus and your body be healthy. It is not a religion – yoga is practiced by a wealth of different cultures. It is simply about helping the body and mind be as healthy as they can be.

Yoga is practiced by Christians, Buddhists, athletes, CEOs, stressed parents, and just about anybody else who seeks calm and focus in their life, along with a healthy body.

Kripalu yoga in particular is a sub-branch of Hatha yoga and traces to an Indian who, in 1965, founded a yoga society in Pennsylvania. He named his practice after his guru, Swami Kripalvananda. The core tenets of this style are gentle acceptance and relaxation.

When you watch yoga on TV or in videos you'll see some styles are wildly energetic or involve extreme contortions. They have practitioners sweating in saunas or exhausted after dancing around for hours. Those are all wonderful styles of yoga – but they aren't what Kripalu is about.

Kripalu is intended to be slow and gentle. It's about developing flexibility and core strength, rather than cardio. Typically in

Kripalu there is no sweating at all. The heart rate is not rising. Instead, it's about relaxation. About gently becoming aware of your body's strengths and capabilities. About slowing down and relaxing. About stretching and developing core strength.

I do recommend also having a cardio aspect to your weekly routine. Each human body needs three main types of exercise – flexibility, strength, and cardio. Kripalu yoga helps you build the first two. Add in some fun cardio activity during other parts of your week, and you'll have an ideal weekly routine to sustain your health for years to come.

ABOUT THIS BOOK

If you have never attempted any yoga before, the best way to learn is from a live human being. That person can see what you are doing with your body and help you do it properly. It's like any three-dimensional motion like learning to play a harp or learning to swim. Developing these skills traditionally involve someone looking at what your body is doing and providing helpful feedback. The more you can get feedback in the early stages, to help you build good foundational skills, the better it will serve you for the decades of your life.

With that being said, not all of us are in a location where we have access to a live human being. In that case, a video is your best second option. Whether it's rented from your local library or watched on YouTube, the video can show you all the three-dimensional movements that your body is making. It is nearly impossible to show those three dimensions of a held pose in a photo. It is practically impossible to properly convey any movement in a photo, even with lines and arrows. A beginner needs to see in motion how the various parts of a body flow.

So for those reasons I wouldn't recommend trying to use a book – either mine or anyone else's – to learn the starting basics of yoga. Yoga is about a body in motion. It's important to understand that motion thoroughly.

This book is intended to help a person who has a basic grounding in yoga to understand my personal routine. I do provide advice about foot placement and balance, but I assume you have been in downward facing dog before. I assume you have a sense of what tree pose is all about. I assume you've been in plank pose and someone has helped you understand what a straight back feels like – or that at least you've done it in front of a mirror and adjusted it for yourself. There are some things it's fairly impossible to guess at without a third-party view of some sort.

I will work on creating free videos on YouTube to go with this free ebook. I will need to get the house clean first, or wait until I can get to a photogenic, warm outdoor location. I'll do my best for you! In the meantime, though, there are a wealth of video options out there for you to learn those basics. I highly recommend you get a mirror or a webcam (just for your own private playback) and practice! Make sure you "watch yourself" somehow so you can see if your alignment looks correct.

Again, the very best option is to have a third party who knows about yoga work with you in the initial stages. Whether it's a free instructor at your local library or a friend who likes yoga, get that feedback as you begin. It will help ensure your practice is safe, healthy, and beneficial.

LISTEN TO YOUR BODY

This book contains my personal sequence I do each morning as a flexibility / core strength routine. I separately do a cardio routine. Flexibility, strength, and cardio are the three aspects of exercise that are good to include in a weekly health plan.

It could be that your flexibility or core strength happens to be less than mine. That when you go into the hurdler's stretch, you cannot press your chest against your forward leg. That when you forward bend you cannot press your palms to the floor. That you can't press your feet flat on the floor in downward-facing dog. That is fine!! We all have different levels of flexibility. Modify the positions so they provide the level of challenge you need.

You should never compare yourself against any other person. Our bodies are different. Our muscles are different! Only focus on your own body. Listen to how it works. Over time you will have different capabilities, as you age and change. That is natural and OK. The sole goal should be as healthy as you can be for the moment. To improve in ways you *can* improve and to be at peace with your body's limitations.

It could be that your flexibility or core strength happens to be more than mine. That in plank you easily hold the pose for two minutes without any arm or stomach stress. That is wonderful! If some of the poses are too basic for you, in my configuration, there are always ways to modify them to add challenge. Look up the options and adjust them to fit your current strengths.

That being said, many of the poses, such as Warrior, are not meant to be "hard." Mountain pose, for example, is not "hard." Rather, it is about becoming more aware of your body. It's about tuning in and learning to listen to all the myriad of messages your body is sending to you. It's about discovering the subtle balance and shift of muscles as you breathe. Hold the pose and simply breathe. Listen. The more you settle into poses like this, the more intimately you come to understand even the slightest changes in specific muscle activity.

ABOUT THE IMAGES

I want this publication to be helpful for people of all shapes, sizes, and colors. With that in mind, I did my best to purchase stock photos demonstrating a variety of yoga practitioners. I selected black models, white models, male models, female models, and so on.

I ran into a challenge, though, in that not all poses were available. Also, I was frustrated that I could only find "model-style" people. Everyone was in quite fit condition and fairly young. I want to show that all ages can enjoy yoga as well as all levels of heaviness.

I will do my best in the coming revisions to add in remaining photos with older people, with heavier people, and with a greater variety of people. If you would like to volunteer for one of the non-photographed poses, please let me know! If you're not a "model" that is fantastic. That's my point. I want to show that *everyone* of all shapes and sizes can do yoga. The more "normal people" I have to illustrate the book with, the better!

SETTING THE STAGE

You can do yoga pretty much anywhere. Sure, when it's nice outside, I roll my yoga mat out on the back porch. I'm surrounded by my container plants and flowers; I bend and stretch where the birds can chirp at me and the butterflies can flutter by.

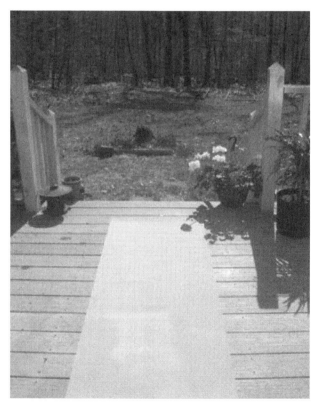

If you're in the city, there could be public parks nearby that are perfect. In the country, your options might be even wider.

In inclement weather, all you need is an empty space to stand. In the winter here are times where I have to push things aside in my kitchen to lay out the mat in a spot just big enough for that mat. That's fine! You do what you can.

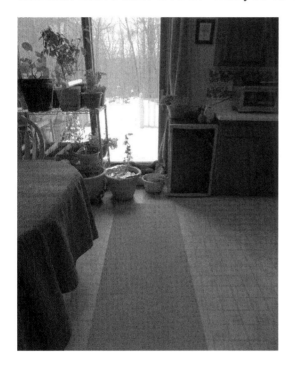

I happen to have a sliding glass door that lets me watch the birdfeeder out back. I fill the shelves here with flowers and plants.

If you don't have a view, that's fine too. You can create the same plant-nook in a tenth-floor apartment. You could even just hang pretty tapestries or inspiring posters in your corner.

You don't even need a rectangle of space. If all you can do is stand in place and use that one spot, that's fine. There are a number of poses like tree pose which will work well that way. There's always a way to get the task done.

You don't even need a mat. You can buy grippy socks that will let your socks have traction on whatever surface you stand on, and go with that.

I do recommend getting a mat at some point, though. It provides a gentle cushion for your hands and feet if you're on a hard floor. If you're on a carpet, it prevents rug burn.

For the purposes of this book, you'll want a yoga mat, a location that lets you lay that yoga mat flat, and a desire to relax. That's it. You don't need any other special devices or objects.

Let's begin!

WHAT TO WEAR

I've done yoga in just about every combination of clothes imaginable. Yoga tops and pants. Sweats. Jeans. Long dresses. Shorts.

On one hand, it doesn't matter what you wear. You can wear anything. Wear what's comfortable so you do yoga. Don't hold off until you get the "right outfit."

On the other hand, it does help to have a top that stays relatively snug against your body. If you do yoga in a loose top, and you bend at the waist, the top might fall into your face.

It also helps to have clothes that move with you. If you are wearing incredibly tight jeans, it could be hard to bend and twist in them.

For your feet, bare feet are best so you don't slip on the mat. If you do wear something on your feet, aim for something grippy so it doesn't slide.

SCHEDULES AND TIME

I strive to do yoga the first thing when I wake up, before anything else. Otherwise I get sucked into tasks and somehow never make time for it. We are all different, in our energy levels and schedules. Whatever works best for you, go for it. Don't worry about "best times" or what other people do. The only thing that matters is that you DO yoga. If it's best fitting in your schedule at midnight, that's good. If it's best fitting at 2pm, that's good too! The most important thing is to do it, not when it's done.

I'm fortunate in that I work from home and set my own schedule. I am able to strive for a full hour of yoga. I find it greatly improves my entire day. My focus is such that I'm able to get tasks done far more quickly after yoga. So the yoga investment "pays back" in increased focus and energy throughout the day. I'm not losing time to yoga – I'm gaining it.

For many people, they have other responsibilities and duties and simply don't have a full hour to spare. That's all right. You can do the full routine more quickly and have it done in a half hour. Or you can leave out items from my normal routine. Whatever works for you, find a way to do the yoga. Even if it's just fifteen minutes. It's better to do something rather than nothing.

Your body will thank you for investing the time!

ADVICE FOR HEALTHY YOGA

Again, always talk with a doctor before starting a routine in order to can get advice on your specific medical situation.

Here are some concepts to keep in mind as you begin a new exercise routine, whether it is my yoga routine here or any other type of activity.

SLOW AND STEADY

In general, no matter what type of exercise you do, avoid "bouncing" into a pose or stance. That bouncing type of motion can over-stretch a muscle. Move into each pose gently and smoothly.

GENTLE HOLDS

Your limbs should not be locked straight and joints should not be over-bent. Keep a slight curve in your elbows. Be loose and relaxed. Be aware of how you are balanced. Put your weight over your knee, rather than forward of your knee to avoid any tilted strain on it.

HYDRATE

Drink ample water to keep your body hydrated as you move. Keep a container of water at your side. A refillable safe-plastic bottle is a good idea, so you can use home-filtered water to drink and simply dish-wash the bottle when you need to. There are flavorings if you don't like the taste of plain water.

TAKE YOUR TIME

There's no race. Go slowly, gently, smoothly, and listen to your body.

This routine here in this book takes me about an hour to finish from start-to-end. That's because I know it and don't have to refer to any notes at each stage. I simply move from pose to pose and hold each one the amount of time that works well for me. I hold a spinal twist until I'm "done" – and I move on.

When you are just starting out, you're going to have to figure out how each pose works and keep referring back to this document to see what to do next. That means it could easily take you an hour just to get through the beginning section. That's all right! If that's the case, work on section two tomorrow and section three the next day. Then cycle through them again.

The more you practice with the routine, the more familiar with it you'll be. The more you'll know how to do each pose without looking it up. The more you'll settle into the pose without having to think carefully about hand alignment or foot alignment. The more you'll move from pose to pose without checking your notes.

It's like any other task in life. Someone who is learning to knit has to give careful thought to the movement of the needles. Someone who's been doing it for a while can mindlessly knit while watching TV. Give yourself time to get comfortable with this new routine!

THE BEGINNING

The beginning is always the settling stage of any exercise routine. You come into it with all sorts of thoughts bouncing through your head. You endure the typical "monkey mind" that all people everywhere have to cope with. The mind leaps from thought to thought with wild abandon. The yoga practice is, in part, about quieting and focusing that mind and training it to gather its energy.

Stand at the center of your mat, facing one of the shorter ends, take a deep breath, and set an intention for this session. It can be releasing stress, forgiving yourself, forgiving someone else, or whatever you wish. It can simply be joy.

Then we begin.

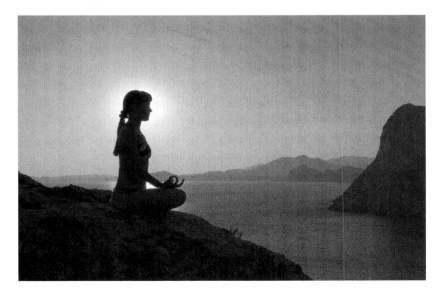

ARMS LIKE COAT SLEEVES

Stand in place with your feet hip-width apart. Imagine that your arms are empty coat sleeves hanging at your side.

Turn your torso as if you are turning to look behind you to the left. Let your arms gently swing with your motion, counter-clockwise.

Now turn your torso as if you are now turning to look behind you to the right. Again, let your arms gently swing, now in a clockwise direction.

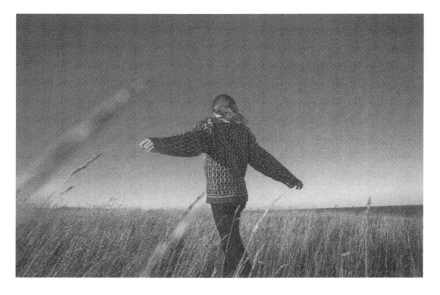

Turn again left. Then right.

Repeat this, slowly, gently, letting your arms flap with the motion. This is a gentle spinal twist, helping to loosen up those all-important cartilage pillows in your spine.

Do this twenty times.

If you aren't comfortable standing or are unable to stand, you can do this sitting on a stool. With every single pose here, you can always modify it. Think of ways to alter it so it works in your situation, and make that version your own.

STANDING CRESCENT MOON

Standing Crescent Moon, or *chandrasana*, is a great way to start bending. Where the previous exercise helped gently twist the spine around its vertical access, this one bends the spine in a side-to-side orientation.

Stand with your feet hip-width apart, with your arms hanging at your side. Raise your arms in a circle up to meet above your head – your left hand going out to the left, your right hand going out to the right. Twine your hands above your head, reaching for the sky.

Gently bend to the left, making a gentle crescent-shaped curve with your body from your toes to the top of your fingers. Your hips sway right and then the chest up to fingers sway left again.

Hold for ten seconds.

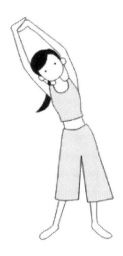

Stand up straight again, and now bend to the right, again making a curve.

Hold for ten seconds.

BACK AND FORWARD BEND

We've twisted our spine vertically. We've curved it left and right. Now it's time to curve it forward and back.

Stand with your feet shoulder-width apart. Put your palms together and reach your hands toward the sky.

Bend back, as if you were going to do a backbend. It's all right if you can only bend back a little bit. The key here is gentle progress. Do what you can.

Hold for ten seconds.

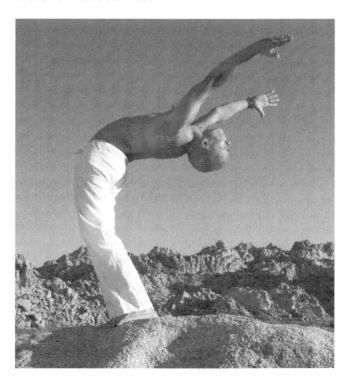

Now stand up straight. Let your hands swing forward in front of you and separate. Have each hand continue its circle down, behind you, and up, coming back around and forward as you bend forward at the waist.

This is *uttanasana* – standing forward bend. Let your hands dangle down before you. Avoid locking the knees – allow them to be loose.

Whether your fingers don't touch the ground, they do, or you can put your palms on the ground, that's all right. Do what you can.

Hold for ten seconds.

I love the forward bend because this is an easy way to see my progress each day. Each day I can bend a little further.

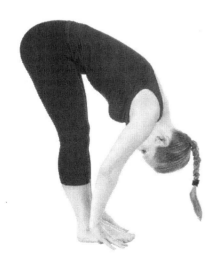

TREE POSE

Tree pose, or *vrikshasana*, is a wonderful pose that is shown all the time in commercials and movies. It is fantastic for building balance which is important for all of us. Especially as we age, the more we can balance, the better our long term health will be.

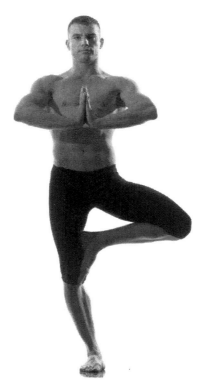

Stand with your feet hip-width apart. Settle into the weight being on one foot. Now bring up the second foot. When you first start doing this, you should probably start with putting the lifted foot against the standing leg's lower calf, just above your ankle.

As you get better at tree pose, and build up your leg muscles, you can work toward putting your lifted foot on the standing leg's thigh above your knee.

Never put your foot on your ankle joint or knee joint. Always aim for muscular parts of your standing leg, rather than joints.

Bring your hands to your chest, touching the palms together.

Hold for thirty seconds.

You'll find when you first start doing tree pose that your sole aim is to not wobble. You're learning about balance. Take deep breaths. Let your mind clear. The more your mind clears, the more settled your pose will be.

As you get better at tree pose, and have the balance part fairly set, think about lifting up in the pose. Imagine you have a string at the crown of your head, like a puppet, and you are being lifted up.

Breathe.

At this point in my years of practice I'm fairly good at tree pose – and even so, if I'm upset about something, I'll be wobbly. One's physical balance is truly impacted by one's emotional turmoil. The better you can settle your emotions and mind, the better health your entire body enjoys.

When the time has passed, put your lifted foot down. Just think about your legs for a minute. Do they feel different from each other? Is one stronger? Is the other one more wobbly?

Then repeat on the opposite leg.

You're now ready to begin sun salutations!

SUN SALUTATION

You've probably heard of sun salutations - *surya namaskara*. In essence this is a sequence of poses that, in one form or another, is part of many yoga routines. It's a good overall stretching routine that ensures most of your important body parts get ample focus and blood flow.

In my routine, the sun salutation is done twice – once starting with the right foot and once starting with the left. You do this entire routine through once. Then you start from the beginning again and do it a second time.

The aim in sun salutations is to do this all as a gentle flow, from one step to another. It's fine at first to keep stopping and referring to these notes. Over time it'll connect together, as you learn the routine.

SKY REACHING POSE

Sky Reaching Pose or *hasta uttanasana* is the start of the sun salutations.

Put your feet hip-width apart near the front short end of the mat, so that most of the mat is behind you.

Start with your hands hanging at your sides.

Raise your hands out to each side – the right hand to the right, the left hand to the left. Continue to circle them up toward the sky. Touch the palms together above your head.

Bend slightly backwards. Stretch up.

Breathe.

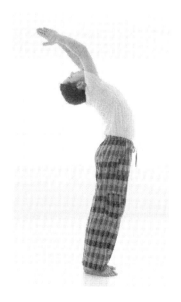

FORWARD BEND

From your stretching-to-the-sky pose, sweep your arms forward and let the palms separate. Let your arms circle down, behind you, up, and then forward as you fold at the waist into a forward bend.

Let your fingers dangle to or touch the floor.

This is *uttanasana*.

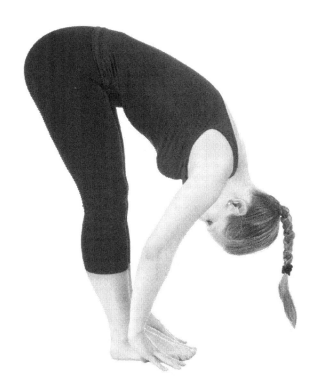

HANDS ABOVE KNEES

This is an interesting pose. It has different names in different styles. Some call it standing half forward bend, or *ardha uttanasana*. Some call it "monkey pose" even though it's nothing like the traditional monkey pose which is a full forward split.

Lift up from the full forward bend and put your hands on your thighs just above your knees. Stretch your back out straight.

Look diagonally forward at the ground before your mat.

I can't even find any good stock images of this pose. This is the best I can do for now, until I can take my own. Keep your hands above your knees, though – you don't want to put pressure on your knees.

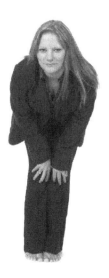

DOWNWARD FACING DOG

Another classic pose - *adho mukha svanasana*. This one builds strength, helps balance, and just feels good once you practice it a while. I know when you're just getting started that it's hard to imagine that poses "feel good." To you, they might feel uncomfortable. But once you start doing yoga for a while, these poses actually feel amazing to hold. It's probably like the joy you used to feel swinging on a swing. It's your body appreciating a motion.

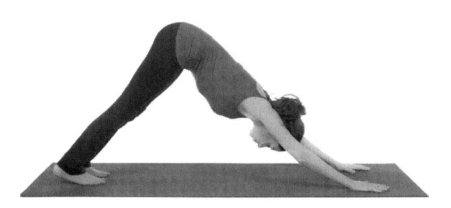

Put your hands on the mat. Step your right foot back first, toward the other end of the mat, and then the left. When you do this the second time through this is where you'd step back with the left foot first, and then the right. Aim to make a triangle shape with your body. You should be evenly balanced on your hands and feet.

It's fine at first if this feels uncomfortable. Your body is using new muscles. Listen to your body and do what you are able to.

Imagine your hips gently stretching toward the sky. Lift up.

Press your heels back toward the mat. Press your hands flat. Roll your shoulders back away from your neck to lengthen your spine.

Once you get better at this, you can stretch one leg up toward the sky and hold for a short while. Then lower that leg and switch to raise up the other leg.

If the soles of your feet don't fully touch the mat at first, that's fine. Try pressing one foot toward the mat, and then switch to press the other foot toward the mat. This is called "walking the dog." Over time your muscles will stretch and you'll be able to do this with both feet fully flat.

PLANK

Plank pose, or *kumbhakasana*, is an amazing pose that is known throughout the exercise and health world. It builds up strong core muscles that are important in daily life.

Move from downward facing dog into plank pose by shifting your weight forward. You should now have your shoulders directly over your hands, and you're on your toes in the back. Your back is fairly straight.

Engage those core stomach muscles.

If you can't hold full plank pose on your arms and toes, you can lower to your elbows as a modification.

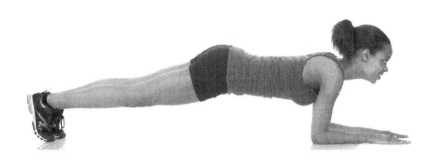

You can also lower your knees to the mat.

Remember, it's fine to modify. Modify away, to suit your current level. Find an alternative that is safe and fits your health and fitness level. We are all different!

COBRA

Cobra – *bhujangasana* - is another great spine-stretching pose. This also feels amazing to me. If it doesn't yet for you, that's fine. Give it time :).

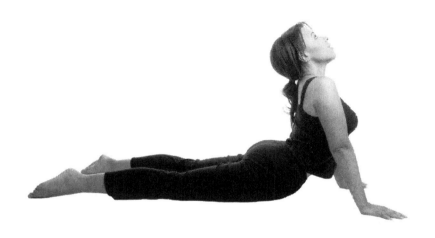

From plank, press your hips down and stretch out your toes. Lift the crown of your head up toward the sky.

Look left and hold. Look straight and hold. Look right and hold. Look straight again and hold.

Stretch your head up.

DOWNWARD FACING DOG

Yup, lift your hips up toward the sky and return to Downward Facing Dog. Your spine goes from curving back to pulling straight again.

This sequence is great for helping your back feel better.

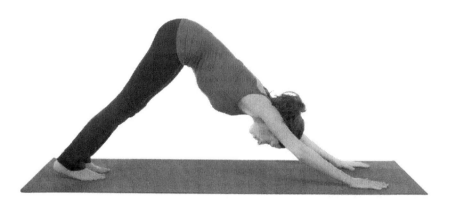

Remember to breathe slowly and deeply with each step. Feel how your body shifts and expands as you breathe.

MOUNTAIN POSE

Mountain pose, or *tadasana*, is simply standing feet hip-width apart. It is a resting pose.

To get into mountain pose, bring your right foot forward to rest near your right hand. Then bring the left one to its side.

If this is your second pass through the sun salutations, bring your left foot forward first, then your right.

Draw to standing, swinging your hands in a circle up over your head as you do. Your left hand goes out to the left and up, while your right hand goes out to the right and up. Your hands will meet palm-to-palm over your head. Bring them down to your chest.

Take in a deep breath.

Take stock of how your body feels.

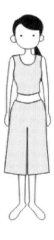

HAND ROTATION

Keeping your thumbs touching, rotate your palms so they face away from you. Point your palms at the floor. Now rotate your palms down so they face you and your fingers are pointing at the floor. Rotate your wrists so the backs of your hands are touching and point your fingers at your chest. Now continue the rotation so your fingers are pointing at the sky.

Lift your hands toward the sky, allowing your elbows to come together briefly as you do. As your hands move up, and separate them.

Make a big vertical circle with your two hands, your right hand going right, your left hand going left. Each one traces half the circle. Then bring them back to meet at your chest.

Repeat.

GATHERING IN

Bring your hands to your chest. Place the palms together.

Press your hands out away from you, to the front. Swing each hand to its side, making a big horizontal half-circle. So the right hand moves outstretched to your right and the left hand moves outstretched to your left. They stay parallel to the floor.

When both hands are fully out at either side, reverse and swing both hands in front of you to meet at the full extension before you.

Draw that in to you.

REPEAT

Go back to the beginning of the Sun Salutation and start again, this time stretching back with the left leg first rather than the right leg.

You are now done with the Sun Salutation portion of the routine. Stand and tune in with your body for a moment.

How does your body feel?

Always check in with your body. Avoid labels like "good" or "bad" – simply listen.

Pay attention.

Understand.

SIDE STANDING SECTION

This is the last section of on-your-feet poses. All of these poses involve being sideways to the mat.

I like positioning my mat so I can look out a side window and watch my bird feeder for these poses.

WARRIOR POSE II

Warrior Pose II or *virabhadrasana II* is another one of those classic yoga poses that you see in commercials a lot. It's a position of strength and concentration.

I do Warrior Pose II as a sequence of related moves, rather than one static pose. So you'll see that this sequence involves a series of motions. It is then repeated with the opposite foot forward.

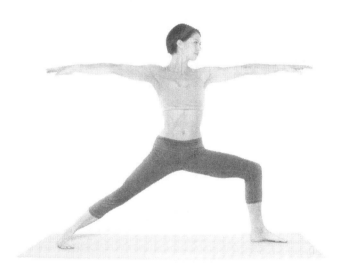

To begin stand sideways on the mat – facing one of the long edges. Stretch your arms out at either side. You're aiming to put your feet about beneath each forearm, just near your elbow. The distance will be different for each of us. You want it to be comfortable and balanced. It's fine to start closer in and to build up to further apart.

Keep your right, back foot with its toes aimed toward the side of the mat. On the second pass, you'll switch so the left foot is the back foot.

Point the left, front foot toward the front of the mat. Lower down so the left leg is bent at the knee. You're aiming for your thigh to be about parallel to the floor, but this might take time to achieve. Ensure the knee stays about over your heel. Do not push your knee forward so it is over your toes – this would cause stress on the knee.

Keep your torso aimed at the side of the mat, then rotate your head so you look forward, as if you are surfing on your mat. Stretch your fingers out, left hand forward, right hand back, and lift through the crown of your head.

Raise up, then settle down into the pose. Raise up a second time, then settle down. Raise up a third time, then balance fully into the pose, equally distributed between both feet. Imagine you are standing sideways in the doorway of double French doors and are balanced on that door-jam between the inside and outside.

Breathe :).

HOLDING THE MOON

Turn both hands so they point palm-up. Imagine that you have a full moon in those arms and curve them slightly to hold the big moon. Then tilt back so that the front hand is pointing toward the sky, tilting the back arm lower to match. Look up at your upper arm.

Hold.

Breathe.

FORWARD REST

Bring your forward left arm down and rest it sideways on your forward left knee, cross-wise. Allow your thigh and forearm to create a plus shape. Raise your back right arm toward the sky.

Look up at your raised arm.

Hold.

Breathe.

FORWARD CIRCLES

Bring your raised right arm forward pointing toward the front of the mat. Then rotate it down toward the floor. Keep going so it points at the back of the mat. Then point it up at the sky again. Continue this rotation for two more rotations.

End with your right arm pointing toward the front of the mat, parallel to the ground. This should give you a long side stretch as you gently pull it forward.

Breathe.

Turn your head so you look into your right arm, with your left ear pointing toward the floor.

Breathe.

Turn your head so you're looking at the ceiling.

Breathe.

LEFT ARM HIGH

Bring your right arm in a circle up and behind you. As you do, raise up so that your left arm is aimed high at the sky, lifting your entire body.

Your right arm should come to rest against your back, right leg.

Stretch up.

Breathe.

TWINING HANDS

Intertwine your fingers behind your back. Still standing tall, press your hands down toward the floor.

Now bend forward at the waist, bringing your torso parallel to the floor. Raise your arms so your hands point toward the back of the mat.

Stretch them back.

MOUNTAIN POSE

Bring your back leg up to be alongside your front leg. Stand in mountain pose and check in with your body.

REPEAT

Go back to the beginning of the Warrior Pose II sequence and repeat with the opposite leg forward.

WARRIOR POSE I

Warrior Pose I, or *virabhadrasana I*, is, as you might imagine, similar to Warrior II.

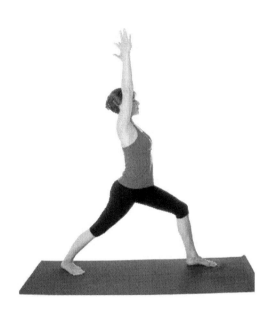

Start again with your feet about two-and-a-half feet apart, or whatever space works well for your proportions, facing the long side of your mat.

Turn your back right foot so it is at a 45 degree angle to the mat. It's pointing diagonally.

Point your front left foot so it points at the short end of the mat.

Rotate your hips so they are also pointing forward at the short end of the mat.

Raise your hands straight up on either side of you, pointing at the ceiling.

Bend your front knee so your thigh is close to parallel to the mat. Again, do not allow your front knee to go past your heel.

Balance so you're equally supported by both feet.

Hold.

Stand and check in with your body.

Now repeat on the opposite side.

INVERTED POSE

Inversions, or being upside-down, are just SO so good for your spine. That's why there are so many inversion tables out there. However, many of the yoga inversion poses like headstands are of course a bit tricky. This is a simpler version for you to try that is fantastic for helping your spine.

Stand with your feet about two-and-a-half feet apart, at the same width we've been doing for previous poses. Have both toes pointing at the long side of the mat.

Stand up tall. Stretch your spine up, for about ten seconds.

Then gently fold at the waist. Let your body hang toward the floor. Let your arms dangle. Let your head dangle. Fold your arms at the elbow and hold them together, to deepen the bend.

Breathe!

In this photo she has her feet a bit wider than I would, but it gives the general idea.

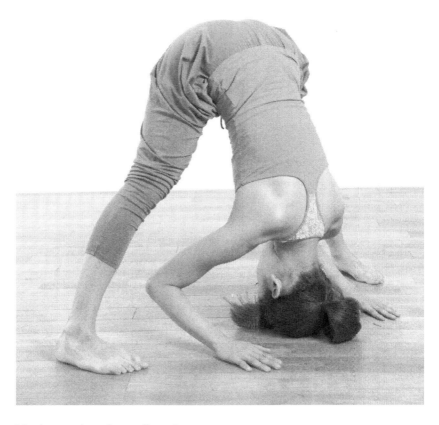

Nod your head yes five times.

Shake your head no five times.

Stand and check in with your body.

You are now done with the standing portion of the routine! It's time to move to a seated position.

MIDDLE SECTION

This section of the routine is all done from a seated or kneeling position. It's good to have a soft mat for this part of the routine. It will cushion you against a floor that might be hard. It will also protect you from a rug-burn-inducing carpet.

A towel will work fine for this part, if you don't have access to a mat.

TUCKED SQUAT

From a standing position, squat down so that your knees are bent and your rear end is a few inches from the floor. You can wrap your hands around your knees if that helps.

Relax.

Give thought to the lower part of your spine. You might feel as if it is lengthening and stretching here. We tend not to think about this area of our body, and it's a fairly important one. Often called the "tail bone," this area is made up of the sacrum and coccyx.

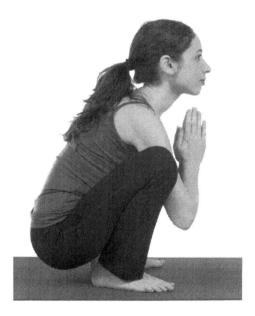

Hold the tucked squat for thirty seconds, giving attentive thought to this lower region of your spine. How is it feeling? Do you get a gentle stretching sensation?

This next image is a public-domain image from Gray's Anatomy, written in 1858. It's a wonderful idea to get a sense of how your spine works. Your spine is so critical to your daily health! While much of your spine involves vertebrae that can move and stretch relative to each other, the sacrum and coccyx are fused. They are connected pieces of bone. But they still have muscles and ligaments around them that can stretch and bend. It's good to take care of these muscles and ensure they work to their best ability.

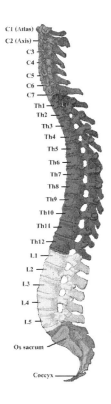

CROSS-LEGGED

Lower yourself to your mat and sit cross-legged. If you can't quite cross your legs, that's fine. Just sit however you can.

Reach your hands high into the sky over your head. Studies show that the arms-above-the-head pose is a "power pose." It can raise your mood and build confidence!

Hold for thirty seconds. Breathe in. Think of a strength you have. Focus on that strength.

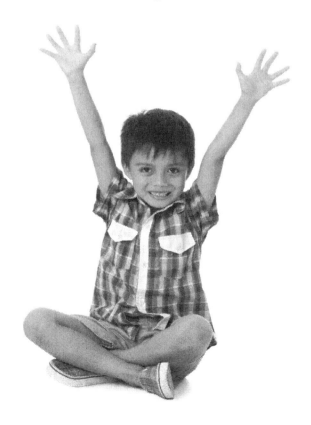

HALF LORD OF THE FISHES

I love this pose. Love love love this pose. It feels so nice to gently twist my spine like this. Again, if it doesn't feel good for you right now, that's fine! You have something to look forward to. For me, this has the same level of pleasure as having a good masseuse find that sweet spot in your aching back muscle and pressing into it. And it's free.

Half Lord of the Fishes is known as *ardha matsyendrasana*.

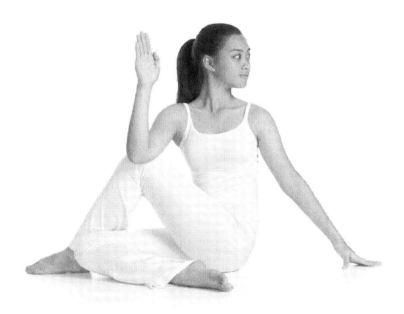

Start by sitting with both legs straight in front of you. Give your right leg a slight bend to the left. You can also leave that right leg straight, if that's easier for you. Bring the left foot toward you and cross it over your right knee.

Bend your right arm at the elbow and point your right hand toward the sky. Put your right elbow against the outside of your left knee.

Now sweep your left arm forward, left, and back, to put it behind you. Follow this arm with your gaze, looking behind you.

Sit up tall, stretching the crown of your head toward the sky.

I know this looks a little complicated but it makes sense when you give it a try. Your spine just feels SO nice being stretched like this.

Hold for thirty seconds.

Repeat on the other side. Since this pose is a bit tricky, I'll list the steps again, with a fresh photo in the opposite configuration.

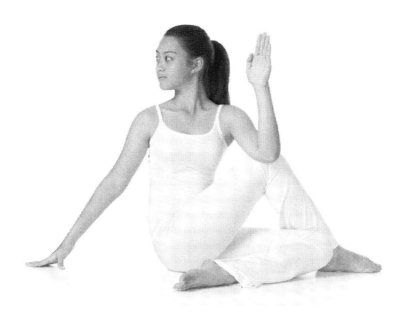

So start by tucking your left leg to the right if you wish, or you can leave it straight. Bring your right leg over to rest your right foot near your left knee. Raise your left fingers toward the sky, bend the left arm at the elbow, and place the left elbow outside the right knee.

Sweep the right arm forward, right, and back, so it is behind you on the mat. Follow this arm with your gaze, looking behind you.

Raise up. Breathe.

CAT AND COW

Another classic pairing of poses. Cat pose is *marjariasana* while cow pose is *bitilasana.*

Get on your hands and knees, facing the front of the mat.

Let your belly sag down, as if you were a cow with heavy udders full of healthy milk for your calf. Raise your rear in the air. Look forward.

Breathe.

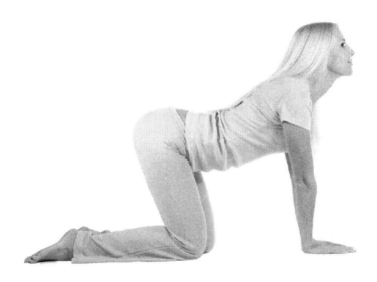

Now arch your back as if you were a stretching cat. Let your head fall down. Breathe.

Repeat this cycle ten times.

EXTENDED CHILD POSE

Extended child pose or *utthita* is a pose of rest. You can definitely use a rest right now!

Let your rear settle back onto your heels. Stretch your hands, palm-down, in front of you. Settle fully down so your chest is close to the mat.

Press your cheek or forehead against the mat, whichever is most comfortable for you.

Hold for thirty seconds.

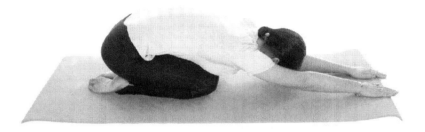

This is the first time that you have a real pause in the routine. At this point you're fairly deep into it and hopefully your mind has stilled a bit. But this is often a spot where monkey-mind begins its activity and starts hopping around.

Breathe. Let the thoughts go. Avoid giving attention to them. Be aware of them, and release them. Don't try to drive them away – that rarely works. Simply acknowledge them and go back to your breath. In. Out.

ROLLING CAT – COW

From extended child pose, shift your weight forward so you are on your forearms. Then up to all fours in cow pose, with your belly sagging. Without stopping, arch up into cat pose. Again, without stopping, ease your rear back onto your heels and stretch in extended child pose.

Roll up to your forearms. Lift up into cow. Arch up into cat. Settle back onto your heels and stretch.

Continue this sequence for ten rounds. This is a moving sequence where you transition from pose to pose without holding. It's a spinal lubrication. Think of your spine curving down, then curving up, then stretching.

End by resting in extended child pose for another thirty seconds.

You are now done with the seated portion of the routine and are closing in on the end! Now you will be doing laying-down poses.

FLOOR SECTION

By now your body should feel fairly nice. At least it does once your body gets used to these moves :).

You are at the restful part of the routine, where you're down on the floor. These poses are mostly about stretching.

HURDLER'S STRETCH

It's important to be cautious when doing a hurdler's stretch. This is a wonderful stretch as long as you're gentle with your knees.

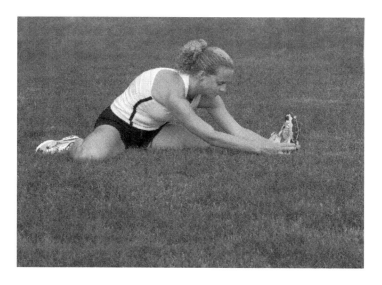

Bend your right knee back and gently stretch your left leg forward. Lower yourself toward your left toes. It's fine if you only go a little way. Avoid locking your left leg straight. This is about a gentle stretch.

Breathe. Hold.

Then lean back toward the back of your mat. Your aim is eventually to be able to lay flat on your back – but again, don't rush. Don't strain. Just let your body gently stretch out.

Repeat on the opposite side, with the right leg forward.

RECLINING SPINAL TWIST

The reclining spinal twist is another pose that I absolutely adore. Some call it reclined Lord of the Fishes (*supta matsyendrasana*) as it is fairly close to that pose. Which I also love :).

Lay flat on your back. Bring your right foot up to sit alongside your left knee. Then fold your right knee to the left, so it points to the left.

Put your arms straight out to either side – the right arm going right, the left arm going left. Put your left hand on your right knee.

Now look to the right, along your arm. Press both shoulders down into the ground.

Breathe.

This feels so good!

Now reverse it, so your left knee is bent and you are looking out along your outstretched left arm.

Breathe.

In this combination photo set of me, called a "multiplicity" photo, the laying spinal twist is the one in the bottom right corner. It shows the second orientation, with my left knee bent and to the right, and my left arm outstretched to the left.

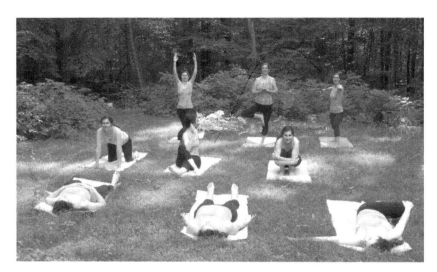

RECLINING GODDESS POSE

Reclining goddess pose is also known as reclined bound angle pose, or *supta baddha konasana*. This is a great hip opener pose.

Lay flat on your back. Bring the heels of your feet up near your pelvis so the soles are flat on the mat and the knees are pointing to the sky. Now put the soles of your feet together and let your knees splay out to either side – your right knee to the right and your left knee to the left.

Bring your arms up over your head, stretched out above you on the mat. Twine your fingers. Bring your fingers toward your head so your elbows also splay out – right elbow to the right, left elbow to the left.

Relax.

DEAD BUG POSE

Dead bug pose or *ananda balasana* is a lot of fun. It encourages you to wiggle!

Lay flat on your back. Lift your legs up and point your soles of your feet at the ceiling. Then lift your arms up and point your fingertips at the ceiling.

Stretch!

Wiggle!

Smile.

Make clockwise circles with your hands and feet. Reverse.

Do scissoring motions with your arms and legs.

Press your heels toward the sky. Then press your toes.

Swing your limbs around.

Release and enjoy.

BRIDGE POSE

Bridge Pose or *setu bandha sarvangasana* is our last main pose we'll be doing. It's also one of my favorites.

Lay flat on your back. Fold your knees so the knees are pointing at the ceiling and your feet are near your rear. Lift up your hips so you have a straight line from your shoulders to your knees.

Bring your hands together beneath your back and intertwine your fingers. Your hands should be about beneath your rear end.

Wriggle your shoulder blades so they're more beneath you to support you. Your weight should be evenly distributed between your shoulder blades and your feet. There should not be weight or pressure on your neck.

Your knees should not splay out to the side, nor should they touch. There should be about a half-foot of space between them. Imagine you are holding a soft foam block in between them.

Hold position.

In this image, she doesn't have her hands clasped beneath her yet.

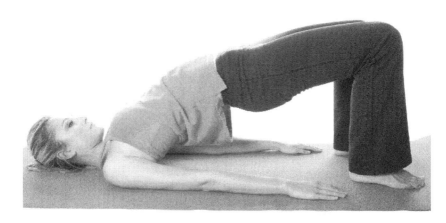

Breathe.

After thirty seconds, release your hands and move them back to your side. Then slowly, vertebrae by vertebrae, lower yourself down. This just feels so amazingly good! Take your time.

One at a time, stretch out your legs. Then lay your arms on either side of you.

Relax.

Breathe.

It is now time for savasana.

SERENITY

We are now at the final stage of the yoga session.

Time to relax and breathe in serenity!

SAVASANA

Normally I call poses by their English names, rather than their Sanskrit names, but in this case with the name being "corpse pose" I would rather call it savasana :). That sounds more soothing and relaxing to me.

Simply lay there. Relaxed. Your feet out. Your arms at your side. Your eyes closed.

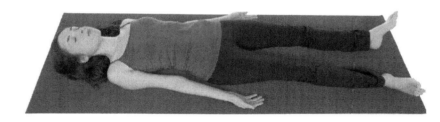

If you tend to get cold, have a blanket or towel to drape over you. This portion of the routine should be calm, relaxing, and quiet.

If thoughts flit into your mind, let them go. Avoid giving them attention. Breathe in.

Breathe out.

Release.

Forgive.

If you tend to fall asleep here, set a timer before you begin for ten minutes.

This savasana provides a much-needed rest after a good stretching routine. It also offers a gentle introduction into meditation.

LOTUS POSITION

Blink yourself aware from savasana. Roll over to your side, then up to sitting cross legged. You can do full lotus position, or *padmasana*, if you wish, where the feet are up on top of the thighs. Do whatever feels right for you.

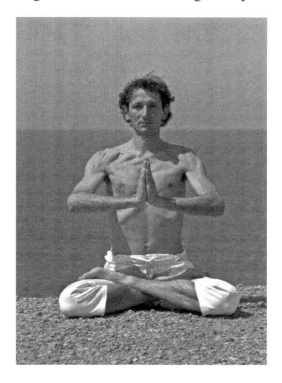

Raise yourself up by the crown of your head, sitting tall.

Imagine there is a golden halo hovering over your head. Gently trace it with the crown of your head clockwise five times.

Then trace it counter-clockwise five times.

Now imagine there is a beautiful orange floating in front of your nose. Trace with your nose clockwise five times, starting at its north pole, then circling down to its south pole and back up.

Then trace it counter-clockwise five times.

Breathe.

NAMASTE

Draw yourself to a standing position.

Bring your hands together at your chest.

Think of all the blessings you have. All the things in life to be grateful for. All those you love.

Then say "Namaste." This means in essence "I reverentially acknowledge you." It is a statement of appreciation.

Namaste.

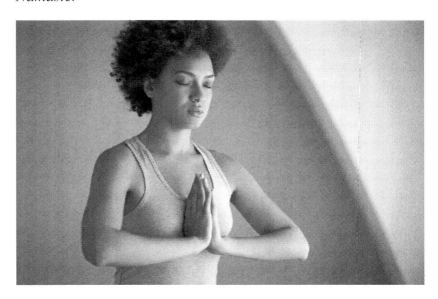

GOING FORWARD

Yoga, like meditation, often creates a myriad of confusing expectations in the mind of a beginner. Maybe they expect monk-on-a-mountaintop serenity at the end of a first session. Maybe they expect the answers to the world's problems to flower in their mind in a kaleidoscope of blossoms.

Probably the one truism is that whatever you go into it expecting, it probably won't be that :). So, with that being said, here are a few thoughts.

Yoga should not hurt. Always listen to your body. If something is hurting, that's a sign that you pressed your current capabilities a little too hard. Ease up a bit. Be gentle with yourself. Always listen to what your body is saying and respect it. You can do a little more the next day, and the next. There is no race. Build your capabilities over time and you'll be amazed how far you get.

Yoga's aim is gentle acceptance. Release any stress about "doing it perfectly" and aim for "doing it the best I can today." Don't judge yourself against experts on YouTube who have been doing this for years. Simply aim to have your own body be a little better than it was yesterday. Think of each session as a curious exploration of where your body is today. Aim for "that's interesting!" rather than "Jeez, why can't I do that?" Breathe deeply. Praise yourself for your efforts.

The first few times that you do yoga it will probably feel awkward and perhaps uncomfortable. You are doing things your body hasn't done before. You are stepping out of your comfort zone. That is all right! That is wonderful. It builds strength in your body, your brain, your lungs, your circulatory system, and many other aspects of you. It helps buffer you against stress and even shore up your immune system.

As you get used to the routine, most people come to think of it as comforting and familiar. The poses will feel good physically. It'll be amazingly wonderful to settle into that spinal twist. Your muscles will sigh with joy as you reach for the sky.

Your brain will ease, too. Stresses will melt away as you settle into the familiar, comfortable poses. You'll forget, for a while, about whatever is pressuring you. Your focus will be the snuggly blanket of motion which you are enveloped in.

It will be like a virtual vacation that can be summoned at any time, in any location. It will be a high-end spa treatment which is wholly free and helps both your body and spirit.

For the beginner, hang in there. All of the benefits are within reach – and they're not that far away.

SUMMARY

We all have so much to be grateful for. We can read and write. Most of us have somewhere warm to sleep at night and food to eat during the day. There are so many people out there who do not have what we have. They could only dream of having the blessings we sometimes take for granted.

Yoga helps us reach this awareness. It helps us reduce stress by realizing just how much we already have. It helps us forgive by helping us see our place in this larger universe we inhabit.

Day by day, yoga helps our health increase, our stress levels decrease, and our ability to help others grow.

Take it one day at a time, and feel free to contact me with questions!

Namaste.

Thank you for reading this *Yoga for Stress Relief and Forgiveness* book! I hope you found some new tools which can help you in your stress relief efforts.

If you enjoyed this book, please leave feedback!

https://www.amazon.com/review/create-review?ie=UTF8&asin=B00S75ILFQ#

You can also post Goodreads and any other systems you use. Together we can help make a difference! The book should be free in nearly all locations. For those where I could not set it to free for some reason, all proceeds of this book benefit battered women's shelters.

If you have a tip I didn't cover, please let me know! Together we can help each other conquer stress.

FREE EBOOKS

I now have 34 free ebooks available on all platforms. If for some reason one isn't free because of a vendor / country issue, the proceeds benefit battered women's shelters.

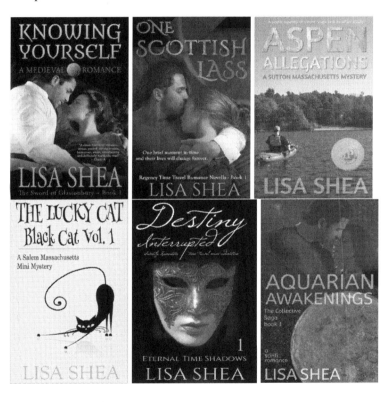

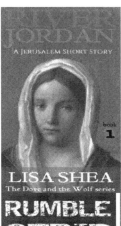
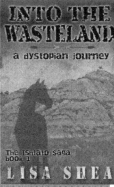
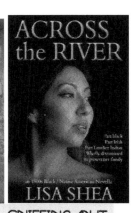
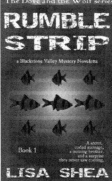
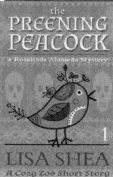
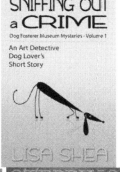
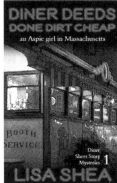
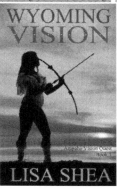
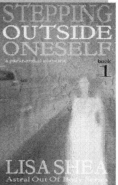

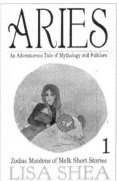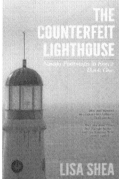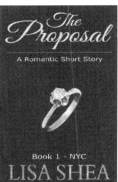
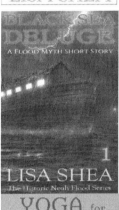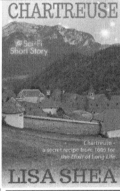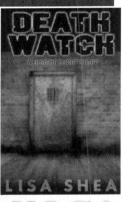
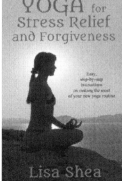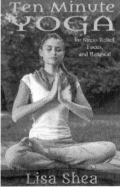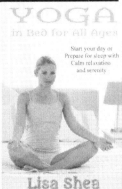

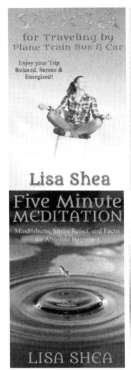 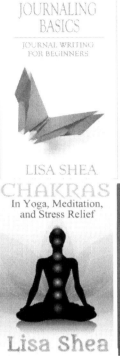 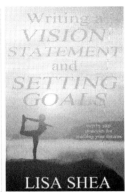 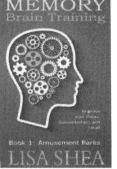

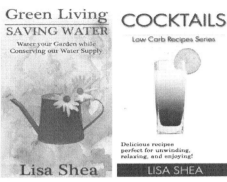
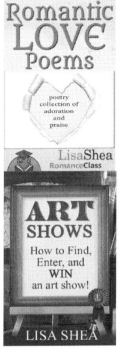

I may have added more free books since releasing this list here. For the most up to date version, be sure to visit:

http://www.lisashea.com/freebooks/

Thank you for supporting the cause!

Be the change you wish to see in the world.

DEDICATION

To Christine, my yoga instructor for many years, whose gentle serenity and warm nature has always impressed me.

To Kripalu, with their amazing staff and supportive environment.

To Elizabeth, Helen, Yvonne, Pamela, Samuel, and Marion who offered specific tips on how to improve this.

To the Sutton Writing Group and Boston Writer's Group, who support me in all my projects.

To my boyfriend, who encourages me in all of my dreams.

Most of all, to my loyal fans on GoodReads, Facebook, Twitter, Google+, and other systems who encourage me. Thank you so much for your enthusiasm!

ABOUT THE AUTHOR

Lisa Shea began her career as a programmer for a number of high-challenge biotech and software companies. After years in the high-pressure industry she decided she wanted to use her skills to help others. She wanted to create a learning environment where those who often have few outlets – stay-at-home moms, those caring for elderly parents, or parents of children with special needs – could reach their dreams and goals.

Through her website BellaOnline.com Lisa strives every day to help every editor and visitor achieve whatever they set out to do.

Please visit BellaOnline.com and see what sites we have open. If one is of interest to you, we'd love to help with training, support, and an encouraging community, so you can reach your dreams!

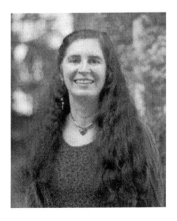

Please visit the following pages for news about free books, discounted releases, and new launches. Feel free to post questions there – I strive to answer within a day!

Facebook:
https://www.facebook.com/LisaSheaAuthor

Twitter:
https://twitter.com/LisaSheaAuthor

Google+:
https://plus.google.com/+LisaSheaAuthor/posts

GoodReads:
https://www.goodreads.com/lisashea/

Blog:
http://www.lisashea.com/lisabase/blog/

Newsletter:
http://www.lisashea.com/lisabase/subscribe.html

Share the news – we all want to enjoy interesting novels!

As a special treat, as a warm thank-you for buying this book and supporting the cause of battered women, here's a sneak peek at the first chapter of *Aspen Allegations*. *Aspen Allegations* is a gentle murder mystery featuring a heroine who loves yoga. Her passion for yoga shines throughout the chapters.

ASPEN ALLEGATIONS - CHAPTER 1

What is life?

It is the flash of a firefly in the night.

It is the breath of a buffalo in the wintertime.

It is the little shadow which runs across the grass

and loses itself in the sunset.

~ *Crowfoot, Blackfoot warrior*

The woods were lovely, dark, and deep. My footfalls on the thick layer of tawny oak leaves made that distinctive crisp-crunch sound that seemed unique in all of nature. The clouds above were soft grey, cottony, a welcome relief from the torrents of Hurricane Sandy which had deluged the east coast two days earlier. Sutton had been lucky. Plum Island, Massachusetts, a mere ninety minutes northeast, had been nearly blown away by eighty-mile-an-hour winds. Here we had seen only a few downed trees, Whitins Pond once again rising over its banks, and the scattering of power outages which seemed to accompany every weather event.

I breathed in a lungful of the rich autumn air tanged with moss, turkey-tail mushroom, and the redolent muskiness of settling vegetation. Nearly all of the deciduous trees had released their weight for the year, helped along in no small part by the gale-force winds of Tuesday. That left only the pine with its greenery of five-needled bursts and the delicate golden sprawls of witch hazel blossoms scattered along the path.

It was nice to be outdoors. Two days of being cooped up in my house-slash-home-office had left me eager to stretch my legs. The Sutton Forest was far quieter than Purgatory Chasm this time of year, in no small part because hunting season had begun a few weeks earlier. The bow-and-arrow set were out stalking the white-tailed deer, and they had just been joined by those eager for coyote, weasel, and fox. I wore a bright orange sarong draped over my jacket in deference to my desire to make it through the day unperforated.

A golden shaft of sunlight streamed across the path, and I smiled at where it highlighted a scattering of what appeared to be small dusty-russet pumpkins. I stooped to pick one up, nudging its segments apart with a thumbnail. A smooth nut stood out within its center. A hickory, perhaps? I would have to look that up later when I returned home. I had finally indulged myself with a smartphone a few years ago when I turned forty, and while I liked to carry it for safety reasons, I preferred to leave it untouched when breathing in the delights of a beautiful day.

The woods were quiet, and I liked them this way. The Sutton Forest network stretched across the middle of the eight-mile-square town, but it seemed that few of the ten-thousand residents knew of this beautiful wilderness. In comparison, Purgatory Chasm, a short mile away, was usually bustling with a multi-faceted selection of humanity. Rowdy teenage boys, not yet convinced of their 'vincibility', dared each other to get closer to the edge of the eighty-foot drop into the crevasse. Cautious parents would climb along its boulder-strewn base, holding the hands of their younger children. Retiree birders would stroll Charley's loop around its perimeter, ever alert for a glimpse of scarlet tanagers.

Purgatory Chasm had an exhibit-filled ranger station, a covered gazebo for picnicking, and a playground carefully floored with shock-absorbing rubber.

Here, though, there was barely a wood sign-board to give one an idea of the lay of the land. The few reservoirs deep in the forest were marked, as well as where the forest proper overlapped with the Whitinsville Water Company property. That was it. Once you headed in here you were on your own. The maze of twisty little passages, all different, were as challenging to navigate as that classic Adventure game where you would be eaten by a grue once your lantern ran out of oil. A person new to the trails would be foolhardy to head in without a GPS or perhaps a pocket full of breadcrumbs.

In the full warmth of summer I would be alert to spot a few American toads, a scattering of dragonflies, and an attentive swarm of mosquitoes. This first day of November was both better and worse. The mosquitoes had long since departed, but along with them they had taken the amphibians and fluttering creatures that I usually delighted in on my walks. I had been rambling for a full hour now and the most I had heard was the plaintive *ank-ank* cry of a nuthatch. Maybe it, too, was wondering where the smaller tasty morsels had gone off to.

Still, with the trees now bare of their leafy cover, there was much to see. The woods were usually dense with foliage, making it hard to peer even a short distance into their depths. Now it was as if a bride had removed her veil and her beauty had been revealed. The edges of a ridge against the grey-blue sky showed a delicate tracery of granite amongst the darker stone. A stand of elderly oaks was stunning, the deep creases of the sand-brown bark rivaling the wise furrows in an aged grandfather's brow.

I came around a corner and stopped in surprise. A staggeringly tall oak had apparently succumbed to the storm's fury and had fallen diagonally across the path. A thick vine traced its way along the length of the tree, adding a beautiful spiraling pattern to the bark. The tree's crown stretched far into the brush on the left, but on the right the roots had been ripped up and a way was clear around them.

I moved off the trail to circumvent this interesting new obstacle in life, eyeing the tree. When I'd parked at the trail head there had been two trucks tucked along the roadside. One had been a crimson pick-up truck with no shotgun racks or other indications of hunting, at least that I could see. With luck the owner was just out for a walk like I was. The other vehicle had been a white F-150 clearly marked as belonging to the Department of Conservation. If the ranger was in here somewhere, hopefully he'd spotted the tree and was making plans to clear the trail. If I hadn't run into him by the time I emerged I'd leave him a note on his windshield.

My foot caught on a hidden root and I stumbled, catching myself against the rough bark of a mature oak. I shook my head, brushing my long, auburn hair back from my eyes. The forest floor was coated with perhaps two inches of oak leaves in tan, chocolate, fawn, and every other shade of brown I could imagine. My usual hunt for mushrooms had been stymied by the dense, natural carpet, and I knew better than to daydream while walking through this hazard.

My eyes moved up – and then stopped in surprise.

The elderly man lay on his back as if he had decided to take a mid-day nap during his stroll. His arms were spread, his head relaxing to one side. But his eyes were wide open, staring unfocused at the sky, long past seeing anything. The crimson blossom at his chest was a counterpoint to the dark green jacket he wore. The blood was congealed, the edges dry.

My hand went into my pocket before I gave it conscious thought, and then I was blowing sharply on the whistle I carried. It was only after a long minute that my mind began to clear from the shock, to give thought to the cell phone I carried in my other pocket. For so many years the whistle had been my first resort, the quickest way to communicate with fellow hikers.

I was just reaching into my other pocket when there was the whir and crunching of an approaching mountain bike. The ranger rode hard into view along the main trail, pulling to a skidding stop at the fallen tree. He was lean and well-built, perhaps a few years older than me, wearing a bright orange vest over a jacket peppered with foresting patches. His eyes swept me with concern.

"Are you hurt, miss?" he asked, his gaze sharp and serious as he caught his breath.

I found I could not speak, could only wave a hand in the direction of the fallen body. The dead man's hair was a pepper of grey amongst darker brown. He had been handsome, in a rough-hewn older cowboy sort of way, and in good shape for his age. Had he slipped on the leaves and fallen against a cut-off tree? Stiff and spindly stumps could almost seem like punji sticks, those sharp-edged spikes that the Viet-Cong laid as traps for unwary infantrymen.

The ranger gave a short shake of his head; I realized he could not see into the ravine from his vantage point. He climbed off his bike; his sure stride brought him to my side in seconds. He pulled up suddenly as his eyes caught sight of the body, then he slid down the slope, moving to kneel at the fallen man's side. He carefully laid a finger against the neck, pausing in silence, but I knew before he dropped his gaze what he would find.

He had his cell phone to his ear in moments, twisting loose the clasp on his bike helmet, running a hand through his thick, dark brown hair. "Jason here. We have a dead body in Sutton Woods, north of Melissa's Path. Just by where I reported that downed tree earlier. Get a team in here right away." He paused for a long moment, listening, his eyes sweeping the forest around him. "No," he responded shortly. "I think he's been –"

There was the shuffling of motion from above; both of us turned suddenly at the noise. A sinewy man stood there in day-glow orange, his wrinkled face speckled with age spots, a visored hunter's cap covering wisps of silvered hair. His eyes moved between the two of us with bright concern. "I heard the whistle. Is something wrong?"

In his hands he held a Ruger 10/22 rifle, the matte barrel pointed somewhere up-trail.

Jason settled into stillness. His eyes remained steady on the older man's, his lean frame solidifying somehow into a prepared crouch. The hand holding the phone gently eased down toward his hip. "Sir, I need to ask you to place your rifle on the ground and step back."

The hunter's worn brow creased in confusion. "I don't understand –"

"Sir," repeated Jason, a steely note sliding into his request. "Put down the rifle." His hand was nearly at his hip now.

The hunter nodded, taking in the patches on Jason's shoulders, and lowered the rifle into the layer of leaves. When he stepped back, Jason moved with a speed I had not thought possible, putting himself between me and the hunter, taking up the rifle as if it was made of bamboo.

The hunter looked between us in surprise, and then his eyes drifted further, drawing in the sight below us. His face went white with shock and he staggered down to one knee. "My God! Is he dead?"

"Have you been shooting today?" asked Jason in response, moving his nose for a moment to the barrel of the gun to sniff for signs of firing.

"Yes, sure, for coyote," agreed the hunter, his voice rough. "But I'm careful! I never would've shot a *person*."

Jason glanced for a moment back at the fallen man. "He might not have been easy to see," he pointed out. "Forest green jacket, blue jeans, he could have looked like a shadowy movement."

The hunter shook his head fiercely. "Ask anyone," he stated, his voice becoming firmer. "I call them my Popovich Principles. I look three times before I even put my finger into the trigger guard. I hear too many tales of accidents. I only took three shots today, and each time my target was solid."

My throat was dry. "Were you sure of your background each time?"

He glanced up at me, and his brow creased even further. "I thought ... but I'm not sure ..."

Jason looked over to me, nodding. "We will figure that all out soon enough," he agreed. "In the meantime, miss ..."

"Morgan," I responded. "Morgan Warren. I live a few miles from here."

"Miss Warren," he echoed, an easing of tension releasing his shoulders. He rested the rifle butt-down on the forest floor. "If you don't mind, we can all wait here for the police and make sure we get all our facts straight."

I settled down cross-legged with my back against an aspen tree, breathing in the scent of juniper, and closed my eyes. After a few minutes a sense of calm resurfaced. The woods drifted toward the peaceful, quiet, eternal sense that it had possessed when I first stepped onto the trail only a short while ago.

* * *

The police had come and gone, the medics had respectfully carried away the dead body, and the forest had eased into a dark blue twilight that resembled the depths of an ocean floor. Jason had remained at my side through it all. Now he stared with me down at the empty space at the base of the ravine. The scattering of witch hazel along the edges added a faint golden glisten to the scene.

"But I didn't hear a shot," I stated finally, as if that made all the difference.

He gave his head a short shake. "Mr. Popovich began his hunting back at dawn," he pointed out. "The victim was apparently shot a few hours later. The body was long dead by the time you reached it. He was undoubtedly dead before you left your house to come here. The M.E. will let us know for sure."

"He looked asleep," I continued. My thoughts were not quite coming in a coherent fashion.

He hesitated for a moment, then put an arm around my shoulder to comfort me. "Can I take you home?"

I shook my head. I was forty-three years old. Certainly old enough to be able to cope with this situation, as unusual as it was. And my home was a mere five-minute drive.

"I'll be fine," I assured him. But it was another long minute before I could pull my eyes from the spot and turn to navigate back around the fallen tree.

"We may need to ask you follow-up questions in the coming days, as we pursue our investigation," he murmured as we made our way up the trail.

"Of course," I agreed, my eyes taking in the forest around me as if it had recently sprung to life. Every twisted branch, every fluttering oak leaf clinging tenaciously to its tree sent a small surge of adrenaline through me. I wrapped my tangerine sarong even closer around my shoulders.

Worry creased Jason's eyes, and he ran a hand through his chestnut-brown hair. I wondered for a moment where his biking helmet had gone, and then remembered the police taking it and his bike back with them at his request.

A strange sense of loss nestled in my heart; I spoke to shake it loose. "I'm sorry to have kept you behind with me."

"Not at all," he demurred with understanding in his eyes. "I was happy to stay."

I lapsed into silence again, absorbed in the soft crunch of leaves beneath my feet, in the soft whistling of the dusk breeze as it scattered through birch and aspen. Jason was steady at my side. My shoulders slowly eased as we walked along the trail.

At last the trail widened before us. I'd never seen the vehicle gate at the mouth standing open, and it brought into focus again just what had happened here. I stared at it for a long moment before bringing my eyes up to the two cars standing side by side, his white F-150, my dark-green Forester.

He fished in a side pocket and brought out a card. "If you need anything – anything at all – you just call," he offered, and his eyes were warm as he handed the card to me.

I nodded, turned, and then I was back in the safety of my car, driving toward the security of home.

Here's where to learn what happened next!

Aspen Allegations

http://www.amazon.com/Aspen-Allegations-Sutton-Massachusetts-Mystery-ebook/dp/B00BO0K7ZI/

Thank you so much for all of your support and encouragement for this important cause.

Made in the USA
Coppell, TX
02 February 2020